Introduction

Dental health is more important than most people realize. And nutrition plays a big role in this. Want to know what to eat to keep your teeth and gums strong?

Our teeth may be small. But they, and our gums, are a lot more important to our health than many of us realize.

Without teeth, we can't chew. Imagine that. No more crunchy raw vegetables and fruits! No more nuts!

Teeth and eating always go together. So, are you eating enough foods good for your teeth? Healthy teeth are one of the best measures of your overall health. With so much confusion about diets and healthy eating, why isn't their focus on dental health? The mouth-body connection is our best way to determine good nutrition.

If you consume too many sugar-filled sodas, sweetened fruit drinks or non-nutritious snacks, you could be at risk for tooth decay. Tooth decay is the single most common chronic childhood

Copyright © 2021 by John Lucas Ph.D.

All rights reserved. No part of this publication may be reproduced, distributed, or transmitted in any form or by any means, including photocopying, recording, or other electronic or mechanical methods, without the prior written permission of the publisher, except in the case of brief quotation embodied in critical reviews and certain other non-commercial uses permitted by copyright law.

Table of Contents

Introduction 3

Dental diet 7

Types of dental and oral diseases 8

Causes of dental and oral diseases 19

Mouth-Healthy Foods and Drinks 26

Dental Recipes 38

Conclusion 124

disease, but the good news is that it is entirely preventable.

Tooth decay happens when plaque come into contact with sugar in the mouth, causing acid to attack the teeth.

Foods that contain sugars of any kind can contribute to tooth decay. To control the amount of sugar you eat, read the nutrition facts and ingredient labels on foods and beverages and choose options that are lowest in sugar. Common sources of sugar in the diet include soft drinks, candy, cookies and pastries. Your physician or a registered dietitian can also provide suggestions for eating a nutritious diet. If your diet lacks certain nutrients, it may be more difficult for tissues in your mouth to resist infection. This may contribute to gum disease. Severe gum disease is a major cause of tooth loss in adults. Many researchers believe that the disease progresses faster and is potentially more severe in people with poor nutrition.

Dental diet

Tooth decay damages your teeth and leads to fillings or even extractions. Decay happens when sugar reacts with the bacteria in plaque. This forms the acids that attack the teeth and destroy the enamel. After this happens many times, the tooth enamel may break down, forming a hole or 'cavity' into the dentine. The tooth can then decay more quickly.

Types of dental and oral diseases

If we don't take care of our teeth and gums, we risk tooth decay, gum disease, and even bone loss.

Meanwhile, the state of our teeth and gums can often signal systemic problems, including cardiovascular disease, celiac disease, diabetes, sinus infection, rheumatoid arthritis, irritable bowel disease, gastroesophageal reflux, alcoholism, and more. In fact, your dentist can sometimes diagnose these conditions before your doctor!

1. Cavities

Cavities are permanently damaged areas in the hard surface of your teeth that develop into tiny openings or holes. Cavities, also called tooth decay or caries, are caused by a combination of factors, including bacteria in your mouth, frequent snacking, sipping sugary drinks and not cleaning your teeth well.

Cavities and tooth decay are among the world's most common health problems. They're especially common in children, teenagers and older adults. But anyone who has teeth can get cavities, including infants. Cavities hurt when they get bigger and touch nerves. An untreated cavity can become a tooth abscess.

If cavities aren't treated, they get larger and affect deeper layers of your teeth. They can lead to a severe toothache, infection and tooth loss. Regular dental visits and good brushing and flossing habits are your best protection against cavities and tooth decay.

2. Periodontal disease

Periodontitis, also generally called gum disease or periodontal disease, begins with bacterial growth in your mouth and may end -- if not properly treated -- with tooth loss due to destruction of the tissue that surrounds your teeth.

Symptoms of periodontitis include swollen or discolored gums, tender gums, bleeding gums, receding gums, change in tooth sensation when eating, loose teeth, tooth loss, and bad breath.

And as if that weren't bad enough, when gums are inflamed and broken, harmful bacteria can enter the bloodstream more easily, leading to other chronic health problems.

Periodontal disease is a risk factor for coronary artery disease. Why? We don't really know for sure, but apparently gum disease doesn't just signal inflammation; it also increases inflammation. And inflammation contributes to coronary artery disease.

Interestingly, the same bacteria that colonize our gums have also been found in arterial-wall plaque.

Even if you don't notice any symptoms, you may still have some degree of gum disease. In some people, gum disease may affect only certain teeth, such as the molars. Only a dentist or a periodontist can recognize and determine the progression of gum disease.

Periodontal disease can be treated with a procedure called root surface debridement. Root surface debridement, which is every bit as much fun as it sounds, involves tools that resemble torture implements, local anesthetic, hours wedged into a dental chair, and a huge bill.

3. Gum disease (gingivitis)

Gingivitis is a common and mild form of gum disease (periodontal disease) that causes irritation, redness and swelling (inflammation) of your gingiva, the part of your gum around the base of your teeth. It's important to take gingivitis seriously and treat it promptly. Gingivitis can lead to much more serious gum disease called periodontitis and tooth loss.

The most common cause of gingivitis is poor oral hygiene. Good oral health habits, such as brushing at least twice a day, flossing daily and getting regular dental checkups, can help prevent and reverse gingivitis.

4.Oral cancer

Aside from the genetic and environmental factors that can influence the development of cancer, certain foods appear to have protective effects against oral cancer, whereas other food products can contribute to an increased risk of developing oral cancer.

Some foods that offer protective effects against oral cancer include green vegetables, carrots, tomatoes, and cruciferous vegetables, all of which provide the greatest benefits when eaten raw.

Certain food products, such as meat, are associated with inducing oxidative damage, which can damage DNA and increase the likelihood of carcinogenesis. Comparatively, foods containing antioxidants such as vitamins A, C, E, beta carotene, and selenium have demonstrated a protective role against oxidative damage and subsequently provided a reduced risk of oral cancer.

Additionally, individuals who consume a diet rich in fat, such as pasta, cheese, red meat, and fried foods, as well as those cooked at high temperatures or in the microwave are at a higher risk of developing oral cancer.

Causes of dental and oral diseases

Your oral cavity collects all sorts of bacteria, viruses, and fungi. Some of them belong there, making up the normal flora of your mouth. They're generally harmless in small quantities. But a diet high in sugar creates conditions in which acid-producing bacteria can flourish. This acid dissolves tooth enamel and causes dental cavities.

Bacteria near your gumline thrive in a sticky matrix called plaque. Plaque accumulates, hardens, and migrates down the length of your tooth if it isn't removed regularly by brushing and flossing. This can inflame your gums and cause the condition known as gingivitis.

Increased inflammation causes your gums to begin to pull away from your teeth. This process creates pockets in which pus may eventually collect. This more advanced stage of gum disease is called periodontitis.

There are many factors that contribute to gingivitis and periodontitis, including:

- smoking
- poor brushing habits
- frequent snacking on sugary foods and drinks
- diabetes
- the use of medications that reduce the amount of saliva in the mouth
- family history, or genetics

- certain infections, such as HIV or AIDS
- hormonal changes in women
- acid reflux, or heartburn
- frequent vomiting, due to the acid
- Diagnosing dental and oral diseases

Most dental and oral problems can be diagnosed during a dental exam. During an exam, your dentist will closely inspect your:

- Teeth
- Mouth

- Throat
- Tongue
- Cheeks
- Jaw
- Neck

Your dentist might tap or scrape at your teeth with various tools or instruments to assist with a diagnosis. A technician at the dentist's office will take dental X-rays of your mouth, making sure to get an image of each of your teeth. Be sure to tell your dentist if you're pregnant. Women who are pregnant shouldn't have X-rays.

A tool called a probe can be used to measure your gum pockets. This small ruler can tell your dentist whether or not you have gum disease or receding gums. In a healthy mouth, the depth of the pockets between the teeth are usually between 1 and 3 millimeters (mm). Any measurement higher than that may mean you have gum disease.

If your dentist finds any abnormal lumps, lesions, or growths in your mouth, they may perform a gum biopsy. During a biopsy, a small piece of tissue is removed from the growth or lesion. The sample is then sent to a laboratory for examination under a microscope to check for cancerous cells.

If oral cancer is suspected, your dentist may also order imaging tests to see if the cancer has spread. Tests may include:

- X-ray
- MRI scan
- CT scan
- Endoscopy

Mouth-Healthy Foods and Drinks

Yogurt and cheeses

Carrots, celery, and leafy greens

Apples

Black and green teas

Lean proteins

Nuts

Why dairy products are good for your teeth?

First, dairy products like cheese, yogurt, and milk encourage your body to produce more saliva, protecting your teeth. Second, cheese and yogurt are high in calcium and protein, which helps strengthen your teeth. Also, yogurt contains probiotics, or beneficial bacteria, for your digestive system. Just remember to choose unsweetened or sugar-free yogurt and add a touch of sweetener or honey yourself. Suppose you are sensitive or allergic to dairy. In that case, you can find calcium- and protein-fortified nut milk like almond, soy, or cashew milk.

Leafy greens

Vegetables should be a star in your diet because they have many health benefits without being heavy or calorie-dense. Vegetables provide vitamins and minerals and help you produce saliva to clean your mouth and keep enamel healthy.

Leafy greens like kale, spinach, chard, or collard greens are full of vitamins and minerals while being low in calories. If you don't go too heavy on the dressings or toppings, you could eat as many leafy greens as you want! Leafy greens are high in calcium, folic acid, and B vitamins, which help your health. You can easily add these leafy greens can to a salad or smoothie.

Why do apples, carrots, and celery help your teeth?

Instead of grabbing a candy bar or dessert, if you have a sweet tooth, eat an apple instead! Apples provide hydration and fiber for your body. By replacing sugary treats with apples, you're promoting good saliva production. Celery helps clean your teeth because the texture can scrape leftover food particles and bacteria away from your teeth.

Carrots and celery are a great source of fiber, vitamin C, and vitamin A. Add raw carrots to a salad, or enjoy some baby carrots as a snack.

Tea, nuts, and lean proteins

Unsweetened black and green teas provide plaque-fighting ingredients. Lean proteins like meat, fish, poultry, and tofu have phosphorous and protein to help keep teeth healthy.

Almonds are great for your teeth because they are a good source of calcium and protein while being low in sugar.

Sugar Substitutes and Sugar-Free Products

Sugar substitutes are available that look and taste like sugar; however, they are not digested the same way as sugar, so they don't "feed" the bacteria in the mouth and therefore don't produce decay-causing acids. They include: erythritol, isomalt, sorbitol, and mannitol. Other sugar substitutes that are available in the U.S. include saccharin, advantame, aspartame , acesulfame potassium , Neotame, and sucralose.

Sugarless or sugar-free food sometimes simply means that no sugar was added to the foods during processing. However, this does not mean that the foods do not contain other natural sweeteners, such as honey, molasses, evaporated cane sugar, fructose, barley malt, or rice syrup. These natural sweeteners contain the same number of calories as sugar and can be just as harmful to teeth.

To determine if the sugarless or sugar-free foods you buy contain natural sweeteners, examine the ingredients label. Words that end in '-ose' (like sucrose and fructose) usually indicate the presence of a natural sweetener. On the label, look under sugars or carbohydrates.

Grapefruit and oranges

While acidic foods can have a negative effect on teeth, grapefruit, oranges, and other citrus fruits can actually benefit oral health when eaten in moderation.

Both grapefruit and oranges contain high levels of vitamin C, which strengthens the blood vessels and connective tissues within the mouth. It slows the progression of gum inflammation that could otherwise lead to gum disease.

Foods to avoid

Poor food choices include

candy -- such as lollipops, hard candies, and

mints -- cookies,

cakes, pies, breads, muffins, potato chips, pretzels, french fres, bananas, raisins, and other dried fruits.

These foods contain large amounts of sugar and/or can stick to teeth, providing a fuel source for bacteria. In addition, cough drops should be used only when necessary as they, like sugary candy, contribute to tooth decay.

Crackers

Dried fruit

Soda

Kombucha

Dental Recipes

1. Basic omelette recipe

Ingredients

3 eggs, beaten

1 tsp sunflower oil

1 tsp butter

Method

STEP 1

Season the beaten eggs well with salt and pepper. Heat the oil and butter in a non-stick frying pan over a medium-low heat until the butter has melted and is foaming.

STEP 2

Pour the eggs into the pan, tilt the pan ever so slightly from one side to another to allow the eggs to swirl and cover the surface of the pan completely. Let the mixture cook for about 20 seconds then scrape a line through the middle with a spatula.

STEP 3

Tilt the pan again to allow it to fill back up with the runny egg. Repeat once or twice more until the egg has just set.

STEP 4

At this point you can fill the omelette with whatever you like – some grated cheese, sliced ham, fresh herbs, sautéed mushrooms or smoked salmon all work well. Scatter the filling over the top of the omelette and fold gently in half with the spatula. Slide onto a plate to serve.

2.Southern Chicken Salad

This delicious low carb salad recipe packs all the flavors of your favorite southern-spiced chicken dish. The heat from the chicken is perfectly complemented by a cooling, yet lightly spiced mayonnaise, a refreshing salsa and a simple yet flavorful salad.

This salad is easily adaptable to suit dietary requirements. Not only is it naturally gluten free, but could be made dairy free by substituting the spicy mayo for a spiced coconut yogurt.

Servings and Prep Time

Serves 2

Time: 35 minutes

Ingredients

For the Chicken:

2 free range chicken breasts

½ a tablespoon of chili powder

1 heaped teaspoon of cayenne pepper

1 heaped teaspoon of ground coriander

1 heaped teaspoon of ground cumin

¼ teaspoon of black pepper

A generous pinch of sea salt

1 tablespoon of extra virgin olive oil

1 tablespoon of coconut oil

For the spicy mayo:

¾ cup of sugar free mayo

¼ cup of sour cream

1 dessertspoon of apple cider vinegar

1 teaspoon of chili powder

½ a teaspoon of cayenne pepper

½ teaspoon of ground coriander

A good pinch of back pepper

A pinch of sea salt

For the tomato salsa:

½ a cup of finely diced cherry tomatos

1 tablespoon of finely diced red onion

1 tablespoon of chopped fresh coriander

1 tablespoon of extra virgin olive oil

1 teaspoon of apple cider vinegar

A generous pinch of sea salt

A pinch of black pepper

For the salad:

½ an iceberg or romaine lettuce

1 avocado sliced or cubed

½ cup of sweet mixed peppers in olive oil

Fresh coriander

You will need:

Two mixing bowls

1 non-stick frying pans

Method

To make the spicy chicken, combine the chili powder, cayenne pepper, ground coriander, ground cumin, pepper and salt in a large mixing bowl. Add the chicken breasts to the seasoning and use your hands to coat both sides of the chicken breasts in the spices.

Add the olive oil and coconut oil to the frying pan over a low/medium heat. Once hot, add the chicken breasts and cook for 15-18 minutes, turning halfway through. Ensure the chicken is piping hot and cooked through thoroughly.

While the chicken cooks you can make the tomato relish and spicy mayo.

To make the mayo, simply combine the ingredients in a mixing bowl and stir to combine. Add more chili for extra spice. Refrigerate until ready to serve.

To make the tomato relish, add the diced tomato, onion and fresh coriander to a bowl. Add the olive oil, apple cider vinegar, salt and pepper and combine ingredients. Reserve in the fridge until ready to serve.

To make the salad simply arrange the lettuce on a large pate or sharing platter. To one side layer the sliced avocado, sweet peppers and fresh coriander.

To serve, slice the spiced chicken and place on top of the salad leaves and dress with the spicy mayo. Complete with a bowl of tomato relish.

3. Healthy Grilled Cheese Sandwich

Grilled cheese made healthier with whole wheat bread instead of white bread and olive oil instead of butter.

Servings: 1

Prep

5 minutes

Cook

4 minutes

Ready in: 9 minutes

Ingredients

2 slices whole wheat bread (preferably fresh)

Sliced Monterrey Jack, Muenster, Cheddar, or Mozzarella Cheese (enough to cover bread)

2 tsp olive oil

Instructions

Preheat a small nonstick fry pan over medium low heat. Place cheese slices (enough to cover bread) between 2 slices of wheat bread. Once fry pan is warm drizzle with 1 teaspoon extra virgin olive oil, slightly tilt pan back and forth to evenly spread oil. Place sandwich in oil, cover with a lid and cook until bottom is golden, about 2 minutes. Then lift sandwich with a spatula an add remaining 1 tsp olive oil to fry pan. Flip sandwich and cook opposite side until golden. Serve immediately.

4. Raw Cashew Cheesecake

With no cooking involved, this cheesecake is incredibly simple to throw together. The key to making this rich and creamy dessert lies in the preparation. The cashews need to be soaked for 4-6 hours in advance, making them lovely and soft.

This will ensure they blend well and create a beautiful silky smooth filling. Vanilla and cinnamon are the key to bringing a little sweetness to this sugar free treat and you may wish to adjust the quantities below according to taste if you would prefer a sweeter dessert With all the richness and texture of a regular cheesecake.

Servings and Prep Time

Serves 8

Time: 10 minutes to prep plus 2.5 hours setting time and 4 -6 hours to soak cashews

Ingredients

For the base:

1 cup of ground almonds

1/2 cup of pecans

3 tablespoons of coconut oil, melted

1 tablespoon ground cinnamon

1 tablespoon vanilla extract

A good pinch of sea salt

For the filling:

2.5 cups of soaked cashews (soaked for 4-6 hours)

1/2 cup of coconut cream

1.5 tablespoons of apple cider vinegar (or more to taste)

1.5 tablespoons of vanilla extract (or more to taste)

1 tablespoon of ground cinnamon (or more to taste)

2 generous tablespoons of coconut oil

A pinch of sea salt

Additional pecans to decorate

You will need:

A food processor

A loose bottomed tin – 6/7 inches in diameter

A mixing bowl

Method

To make the cheesecake base, add the whole pecans to a food processor and pulse until the texture is crumbly but not too fine. This will add a bit of crunch to the base. Pour the melted coconut oil into a mixing bowl and add the ground pecans, ground almonds, cinnamon, vanilla and salt. Stir thoroughly to combine, but don't overwork the mixture. Pour this into the loose bottomed tin and press into a flat and even layer to form the base. Place this in the fridge to set while you make the filling.

5. Mushroom Asparagus Frittata

The key to making the perfect frittata is in the balance of flavor and allowing the flavor of the veggies and herbs to infuse in the pan before adding the egg mixture. Ensure also that you give the eggs a really good whisk before adding to the pan to allow for a nice fluffy texture.

This low carb recipe is not only packed with taste and healthy fats, but is also gluten free, with the option of being dairy free too.

Servings and Prep Time

Serves 6-8

Time: 30 minutes including prep

Ingredients

8 medium eggs

2 cups of sliced chestnut mushrooms

5 large asparagus spears

1 red onion cut into small wedges

1 generous tablespoon of grass fed butter or coconut oil

5 sprigs of fresh rosemary

A generous pinch of sea salt

A generous pinch of black pepper

Optional: sliced goats cheese

You will need:

A large oven proof non stick frying pan

A small saucepan

A large mixing bowl

Method

Preheat the oven to 180 degrees for fan assisted, 200 degrees for conventional, 400 degrees F, or gas mark 6.

Begin by adding the asparagus spears to a small pan of boiling water. Allow to boil for 3 minutes – just enough to allow the asparagus to become tender.

In the meantime, melt the butter or oil in a large non stick frying pan over a medium heat. Add the onion wedges and rosemary. Fry gently for four minutes until the onion begins to soften.

Add the mushrooms and asparagus to the pan and continue to fry for a further 2 minutes until tender.

While the vegetables are cooking, crack the eggs into a large mixing bowl and season generously with salt and pepper. Beat the eggs with a whisk until thoroughly combined.

Remove the rosemary from the pan. Turn the heat up slightly and pour the egg mixture straight over the vegetables, tilt the pan to ensure the egg mixture completely surrounds the vegetables.

Allow this to cook for 2-3 minutes until part set. You will see the egg begin to set around the edges of the pan and towards the center.

Add the slices of cheese to the surface of the frittata.

Transfer the pan to the oven and bake for 10-12 minutes until completely set and the cheese is bubbling.

The frittata tastes delicious both hot and cold served with salad or steamed vegetables.

Transfer to an airtight container for storage and refrigerate. This will keep in the fridge for up to 3 days.

6. Italian Sandwich Roll-Ups

Italian Sandwich Roll-ups – The perfect combination of meats, cheeses, and veggies. These roll ups are full of flavor and always a crowd pleaser. I'm warning you now, they will go fast

Ingredients

8 tortillas

8 ounces cream cheese, softened

1 tablespoon Italian seasoning

1/4 cup banana peppers, chopped

1/4 cup roasted red peppers, chopped

24 slices Genoa salami

24 slices of ham

1 pack pepperoni (about 32 small slices)

16 slices Provolone cheese

2 large tomatoes, thinly sliced (remove some of the juice and seeds)

1 head of lettuce

Instructions

In medium bowl, combine cream cheese, banana peppers, roasted red peppers, and Italian seasoning. Mix with spoon until all ingredients are well combined.

Spread about three tablespoons of cream cheese mixture onto a tortilla.

On top of the cream cheese mixture, place three slices of salami, three slices of pepperoni, three slices of ham, and three slices of Provolone cheese, leaving about 1/2-inch border around the edge.

Top with two slices of tomato and a few pieces of lettuce. Roll tortilla up tightly.

Place toothpicks about 1-inch apart down the rolled tortilla. Cut in between the toothpicks to create pinwheels.

Repeat with remaining tortillas and fillings. Serve immediately or refrigerate until you're ready to serve sandwiches.

7. Light and Creamy Apple Salad

Ingredients

2 cups diced, unpeeled Granny Smith or Golden Delicious apples (about 1.5 medium apples)

2 cups diced unpeeled red apples (such as Red Delicious, Gala, or Honey Crisp) (about 1.5 medium apples)

¼ cup golden raisins

1 tablespoon apple juice (or sub with orange juice or lemon juice)

5.3 ounces (about ½ cup) Greek-style vanilla yogurt can substitute with plain Greek yogurt and a dash of vanilla extract if you prefer a less-sweet option

¼ cup light mayonnaise

½ teaspoon apple pie spice (can substitute with ¼ teaspoon cinnamon and ¼ teaspoon of nutmeg)

¼ cup chopped toasted pecans

¼ cup unsweetened shredded coconut

Instructions In a medium bowl, toss together apples, raisins, and juice.

In a small bowl, whisk together yogurt, mayonnaise and apple pie spice.

Gently combine yogurt mixture with apple mixture. Refrigerate until ready to serve.

Just before serving, sprinkle with pecans and coconut.

Notes

Prep Ahead! This apple salad stays fresh in an airtight container in the refrigerator for at least 2 days. Just wait to add the nuts and coconut on top until you're ready to serve.

Recipe Variations:

Make this apple salad with about ½ cup diced celery -- it will be like a Waldorf Salad!

Substitute with other types of nuts like almonds, peanuts, hazelnuts or cashews

Dried cranberries are a great substitute for the raisins

Lemon or orange zest would add a stronger, brighter citrus flavor to the dish

Nutrition

Serving: 1/8 of the salad | Calories: 124kcal | Carbohydrates: 17g | Protein: 2g | Fat: 6g | Saturated Fat: 2g | Cholesterol: 1mg | Sodium: 60mg | Potassium: 153mg | Fiber: 2g | Sugar: 12g | Vitamin A: 35IU | Vitamin C: 3.3mg | Calcium: 9mg | Iron: 0.4mg

8. Hot and Sour King Prawn Soup

The beauty of this soup is in its simplicity and versatility. If you prefer a little extra heat, you can add extra chilies to your taste. For more of that vibrant tang, add another tablespoon of cider vinegar. Perfect paleo dinner! A flavorful low carb lunch or a sublimely simple dinner party entrée.

Servings and Prep Time

Serves 2

Time: 20 minutes

Ingredients

150g uncooked king prawns

1 cup of sliced chestnut mushrooms

1 thumb sized piece of peeled and sliced fresh ginger

3 fresh green chilies, sliced

1 clove of finely sliced garlic

3 sliced spring onions

2 tablespoons of apple cider vinegar

2 tablespoons of sesame oil

750 ml of hot chicken stock

A generous pinch of black pepper

A handful of fresh coriander to serve

You will need:

A large heavy bottomed casserole dish

Method

Add the sesame oil to the casserole dish over a low heat. Once hot, add the sliced mushrooms and cook gently for 3 minutes. Add the garlic, chilies, ginger and black pepper and continue to cook in the oil for a further 1-2 minutes, stirring regularly. Pour the apple cider vinegar into the pan and give all the ingredients a good stir.

Add the hot chicken stock to the casserole dish, and bring the soup to a gentle boil.

Add the king prawns and allow to simmer gently for 10 minutes until the prawns are pink and cooked through.

Scatter the chopped fresh coriander and spring onions over the soup to serve.

9. Homemade Spaghetti Os

Ingredients

16 oz tomato sauce*

2 Tbsp tomato paste

1/4 tsp garlic powder

1/4 tsp paprika

1/4 tsp onion powder

1/8 tsp dried thyme (optional)

1/2 tsp salt

1 Tbsp honey (optional)

6 Tbsp milk

2 Tbsp butter

1 cup packed cheddar cheese, shredded (about 5 oz)

2 cups small pasta, about 8 oz (ditalini if you're shopping in store, or anelletti for the traditional O-shaped noodles)*

additional salt, to taste

Instructions

Start with the pasta and cook, on medium-high, al dente, according to the directions on the package, stirring occasionally.

Meanwhile, combine tomato sauce, tomato paste, spices, milk and butter in a saucepan and bring to a simmer. The honey is optional but adds the signature "sweet" taste that you're used to in spaghetti O's. If you add it, add it with the milk and butter.

Add cheese and stir until melted. Turn heat to low until pasta is done.

Strain pasta when done and portion into serving bowls.

Ladle finished sauce over pasta, adding more sauce for those who like it saucy!

Notes

* You can substitute fresh tomatoes, canned whole tomatoes or canned diced tomatoes for the tomato sauce. You can even use leftover tomato basil soup or pizza sauce. If you're using whole or diced tomatoes, puree first and then measure.

* If you use another pasta that is slightly larger, like small shells or macaroni, you might need to increase the quantity.

9. Granola Recipe: Cinnamon Crunch

The key to getting the granola just right is to not pulse it for too long in the food processor – this will ensure you have good sized clusters of nuts and seeds that bake evenly. Equally important is to turn the granola at regular intervals during baking.

The beauty of this recipe is that you can play about with the ingredients and use different nuts and seeds and adjust the sweetness to your personal taste.

Servings

5 serves

Ingredients

1 cup of almonds

1 cup of pecans

½ cup of cashews

1 cup of dessicated coconut

¼ cup of coconut flakes

¼ cup of pumpkin seeds

¼ cup of sunflower seeds

1.5 tablespoon of ground cinnamon (add more to taste)

1 tablespoon of unsweetened almond or cashew butter

1 tablespoon of coconut oil

1 teaspoon of vanilla extract or powder

A pinch of sea salt

You will need:

A food processor

A large baking tray

Baking paper

A mixing bowl

A small saucepan

Method

Preheat the oven to 180 degrees for fan assisted. 200 degrees for conventional, 400 degrees F, or gas mark 6.

Line a large baking tray with a sheet of baking paper.

Add the almonds, pecans and cashew nuts to the food processer. Pulse briefly to break the nuts into chunks.

Add the nut butter, coconut oil and cinnamon to a small saucepan over a low heat. As the coconut oil and almond butter begin to melt, stir continuously to ensure all the ingredients are thoroughly combined.

Transfer the nut mixture from the food processor to the mixing bowl and add the pumpkin seeds, sunflower seeds, desiccated coconut, coconut flakes, vanilla extract and salt. Stir thoroughly to combine.

Pour the liquid mixture over the nuts and seeds and stir thoroughly, ensuring the granola mix is evenly covered.

Tip the mixture out onto the lined baking tray and spread the granola out in an even layer.

Place in the center of the oven to bake for 20 – 25 minutes turning frequently to ensure an even bake.

Remove the granola from the oven and allow to cool completely before serving with ice cold nut milk!

Transfer to an airtight container for storage.

10. Taco Pasta Salad

This taco pasta salad is such a yummy dish, and its perfect for a spring or summer potluck or bbq! It makes a lot, so its great for a big family gathering! But the recipe can also be easily cut in half if you don't need to feed quite as many hungry bellies.

It's also a great dish because you can customize it. If someone does't like bell pepper leave it out, if you want more protein, add in some black beans, etc.

Ingredients

16 oz rotini pasta (or other medium sized noodle)

1 lb ground beef

3 TBS taco seasoning

1.5 cups chopped tomatoes

1 cup diced green bell pepper

2-3 cups Mexican Style Shredded Cheese

4 cups shredded lettuce (you can buy this already shredded at some stores)

15 oz French Dressing

3 cups slightly crushed nacho cheese or tortilla chips

chopped cilantro (optional)

Instructions

Bring a large pot of water to boil. Cook rotini noodles according to package directions. Rinse off in cold water.

In a large skillet, cook ground beef. Drain grease.

Mix in taco seasoning.

In a large bowl add pasta, ground beef, tomatoes, bell pepper, cheese, and lettuce.

Pour French Dressing over the top.

Stir everything together.

Cover and place in fridge if you're not ready to serve yet.

When ready to serve add in crushed chips (so they don't get soggy).

Top with chopped cilantro if desired.

Nutrition

Calories: 592kcal | Carbohydrates: 55g | Protein: 16g | Fat: 34g | Saturated Fat: 8g | Cholesterol: 34mg | Sodium: 677mg | Potassium: 360mg | Fiber: 3g | Sugar: 7g | Vitamin A: 465IU | Vitamin C: 11.3mg | Calcium: 196mg | Iron: 2.1mg

11. Chipotle Black Bean Tortilla Soup

This chipotle black bean vegetarian tortilla soup is quick, easy, and full of bright Mexican flavors. Enjoy it as-is, or top with the works for a fun and flavor-packed meatless meal.

Ingredients

4-6 small corn tortillas

olive or avocado oil

kosher salt

1 large yellow or sweet onion chopped

2 tablespoons tomato paste

1 tablespoon adobo sauce optional, see note

1 tablespoon chili powder

2 teaspoons oregano Mexican oregano if you have it

1 teaspoon garlic powder

1 teaspoon ground cumin

1 (28 ounce) can diced tomatoes fire-roasted if possible

4 cups vegetable stock or broth

1 (15 ounce) can black beans drained and rinsed

1 (15 ounce) can pinto beans drained and rinsed

1 cup frozen corn kernels

1 teaspoon fresh lime juice

avocado, sour cream, Cotija cheese, cilantro, etc. as desired, for serving

Instructions

Make tortilla strips (optional). Preheat oven to 375 degrees F. Brush each tortilla lightly with olive or avocado oil on both sides. Using a chef's knife or a pizza cutter, slice tortillas in half, then into thin strips. Place the strips on a baking sheet and bake for 10 to 12 minutes until crispy and lightly browned. Sprinkle with kosher salt and set aside. (This can be done 1-2 days in advance; store in an airtight container at room temperature.)

Make the soup. Warm 2 teaspoons oil in a large stockpot or Dutch oven over medium-high heat. Add onion and cook 2-3 minutes, until it begins to soften. Stir in tomato paste, adobo sauce (if using), chili powder, oregano, garlic powder, and cumin. Cook for about 1 minute, stirring well.

Add diced tomatoes. Cook 2-3 minutes, stirring occasionally, until the tomato juices reduce and thicken a bit.

Stir in stock, beans, and corn. Bring soup to a simmer, then reduce heat to low and cook 12-15 minutes.

Finish and serve. Add a squeeze of lime juice. Taste the soup and add a bit of extra salt if desired. Serve as desired with tortilla crisps, avocado, sour cream, Cotija, fresh cilantro, etc.

Nutrition Estimate

calories: 283kcal, carbohydrates: 53g, protein: 15g, fat: 2g, saturated fat: 1g, sodium: 1463mg, potassium: 726mg, fiber: 15g, sugar: 7g, vitamin a: 1363iu, vitamin c: 6mg, calcium: 119mg, iron: 5mg

12. Low Carb Chicken Alfredo Bake Recipe

The beauty of this sauce is that once you have perfected the garlic, cream and cheese sauce as a base, you can add any low carb vegetables of your choice.

Quick and easy to make

Servings and Prep Time

Serves 6

Time: 1 hr including prep

Ingredients

500g diced chicken breast

1 teaspoon of dried oregano

1 teaspoon of dried thyme

A generous pinch of sea salt

A generous pinch of black pepper

1 tablespoon of extra virgin olive oil

8 Stems of broccolini

2 tablespoons of full fat butter

2 tablespoons of extra virgin olive oil

1 finely sliced red onion

2 cloves of minced garlic

2 cups of mushrooms

2.5 cups of thick cream

1/2 cup grated parmesan

A generous pinch of sea salt

A generous pinch of black pepper

3/4 cup mozzarella sliced

You will need:

A mixing bowl

A large non stick pan

A baking dish approx 9 x 9 inches wide

Method

Pre-heat the oven to 180 degrees for fan assisted, 200 for conventional, 400 degrees F or gas mark 6.

Add the diced chicken, oregano, thyme, salt and pepper to a mixing bowl. Use your hands to mix thoroughly, ensuring the chicken is well coated in the seasoning. Heat one tablespoon of olive oil in a large non stick pan over a medium heat. Fry the chicken gently until cooked through. Remove from the pan and lay across the base of the baking dish.

While the chicken is frying, add the broccolini to a pan of boiling water and simmer until firm but tender – around 4 minutes. Drain and add to the baking dish with the chicken.

13. Vegetable Fried Rice

Ingredients

1 ½ teaspoons + 2 tablespoons avocado oil or safflower oil, divided

2 eggs, whisked together

1 small white onion, finely chopped (about 1 cup)

2 medium carrots, finely chopped (about ½ cup)

2 cups additional veggies, cut into very small pieces for quick cooking (see photos for size reference; options

include snow peas, asparagus, broccoli, cabbage, bell pepper, and/or fresh or frozen peas—no need to thaw first)

¼ teaspoon salt, more to taste

1 tablespoon grated or finely minced fresh ginger

2 large cloves garlic, pressed or minced

Pinch of red pepper flakes

2 cups cooked brown rice (*see notes!)

1 cup greens (optional), such as spinach, baby kale or tatsoi

3 green onions, chopped

1 tablespoon reduced-sodium tamari or soy sauce**

1 teaspoon toasted sesame oil

Chili-garlic sauce or sriracha, for serving (optional)

Instructions

This recipe comes together quickly. Before you get started, make sure that all of your ingredients are prepped and within an arm's reach from the stove. Also have an empty bowl nearby for holding the cooked eggs and veggies.

I'm suggesting that you start over medium-high heat, but if at any point you catch a whiff of oil or food burning, reduce the heat to medium.

Warm a large cast iron or stainless-steel skillet over medium-high heat until a few drops of water evaporate within a couple of seconds. Immediately add 1 ½ teaspoons of oil and swirl the pan to coat the bottom. Add the scrambled eggs and swirl the pan so they cover the bottom. Cook until they are just lightly set, flipping or stirring along the way. Transfer the eggs to a bowl and wipe out the pan with a heat-proof spatula.

Return the pan to heat and add 1 tablespoon of oil. Add the onion and carrots and cook, stirring often, until the onions are translucent and the carrots are tender, about 3 to 5 minutes.

Add the remaining veggies and salt. Continue cooking, stirring occasionally (don't stir too often, or the veggies won't have a chance to turn golden on the edges), until the veggies are cooked through and turning golden, about 3 to 5 more minutes. In the meantime, use the edge of your spatula or a spoon to break up the scrambled eggs into smaller pieces.

Use a big spatula or spoon to transfer the contents of the pan to the bowl with the cooked eggs. Return the pan to heat and the remaining 1 tablespoon oil. Add the ginger, garlic and red pepper flakes, and cook until fragrant while stirring constantly, about 30 seconds. Add the rice and mix it all together. Cook, stirring occasionally, until the rice is hot and starting to turn golden on the edges, about 3 to 5 minutes.

Add the greens (if using) and green onions, and stir to combine. Add the cooked veggies and eggs and stir to combine. Remove the pan from the heat and stir in the tamari and sesame oil. Taste, and add a little more tamari if you'd like more soy flavor (don't overdo it or it will drown out the other flavors) or salt, if the dish needs an extra boost of overall flavor.

Divide into bowls and serve immediately. I usually serve mine with chili-garlic sauce or sriracha on the side. Leftovers store well in the refrigerator, covered, for 3 to 4 days (if you used purple cabbage, it might stain your scrambled eggs a funny blue color, but it's fine to eat).

14. Cabbage Slaw Salad Recipe

This low carb, full fat slaw is so quick and easy to make. It is the perfect side for BBQ meats, used as a gluten free burger relish or even to accompany freshly roasted chicken!

The key to making the perfect slaw is to slice the cabbage as finely as possible and ensure an even coating of the dressing.

The sour cream and mayonnaise creates a beautifully rich and creamy base offset by the tang of apple cider vinegar and hot mustard. Once you have created your creamy dressing, you can always adjust the seasonings below to your own personal taste or experiment with alternative low carb vegetables.

Servings and Prep Time

Serves 4

Time: 10 minutes

Ingredients

2 cups of finely sliced red cabbage

2 cups of finely sliced white cabbage

½ a red onion, finely diced

½ cup sour cream

½ cup sugar free mayonnaise

1 tablespoon of apple cider vinegar

1 tablespoon of Dijon mustard

1 teaspoon celery salt

1 teaspoon ground cumin

¼ teaspoon of black pepper

A good pinch of sea salt

You will need:

Two mixing bowls

Method

Add the red cabbage, white cabbage and red onion to a large mixing bowl and place to one side.

In a separate bowl, add the apple cider vinegar, sour cream, mayonnaise, mustard, celery salt, cumin, salt and pepper. Mix together thoroughly to combine all ingredients.

Add the cabbage and onion mixture to the dressing and stir to combine, ensuring the cabbage and onion is evenly coated in the mixture.

Serve with salad or as an accompaniment to meat.

Store in the fridge in an airtight container.

15. Five-Way Mini Meatloaves

Ingredients:

Base Meatloaf Recipe:

1-1/2 pounds Ground Beef (93% lean or leaner)

1/3 cup saltine, butter cracker crumbs or Panko bread crumbs

1/3 cup finely chopped onion

1/3 cup reduced-fat 2% milk

1 egg, lightly beaten

1 teaspoon minced garlic

1/2 teaspoon salt

1/4 teaspoon pepper

Cooking:

Heat oven to 350°F. Combine all ingredients in large bowl, mixing lightly but thoroughly.

Cook's Tip: To make cracker crumbs, place crackers in food-safe plastic bag;

close bag securely, squeezing out air. Crush crackers with rolling pin to form fine crumbs.

Shape beef mixture into 12 equal portions. Place into 12-cup standard muffin pan, lightly patting beef mixture to level top. Bake in 350°F oven 19 to 20 minutes, until internal temperature reaches 160°F.

Cook's Tip: Cooking times are for fresh or thoroughly thawed Ground Beef. Ground Beef should be cooked to an internal temperature of 160°F. Color is not a reliable indicator of Ground Beef doneness.

Remove from oven. Garnish with Toppings, as desired. Let stand 5 minutes before serving.

Recipe Variations:

Italian Mini Meatloaves: Add 1/2 cup chopped mushrooms, 1/2 cup pasta sauce and 1/4 cup chopped fresh basil to base meatloaf ingredients. Bake 22 to 24 minutes, until internal temperature reaches 160°F. Evenly top with shredded Parmesan cheese. Let stand 5 minutes before serving. Serve with additional pasta sauce and garnish with additional chopped basil, as desired.

Greek Mini Meatloaves: Add 3 tablespoons chopped Kalamata olives and 1/2 teaspoon dried oregano to base meatloaf ingredients. Bake 22 to 24 minutes, until internal temperature reaches 160°F. Evenly top with crumbled feta cheese. Let stand 5 minutes before serving. Serve with prepared tzatiki sauce. Garnish with sliced cucumber, as desired.

Asian Mini Meatloaves: Add 1/4 cup chopped green onions and 1 teaspoon minced fresh ginger to base meatloaf ingredients. Bake 22 to 24 minutes, until internal temperature reaches 160°F. Evenly top with hoisin sauce or teriyaki glaze. Let stand 5 minutes before serving. Garnish with chopped peanuts, sliced green onions or chopped cilantro, as desired.

Spanish Mini Meatloaves: Add 1/2 cup finely chopped red bell pepper, 1/4 cup chopped Spanish olives and 1 teaspoon smoked paprika to base meatloaf ingredients. Bake 22 to 24 minutes, until internal temperature reaches 160°F. Evenly top with shredded manchego cheese. Let stand 5 minutes before serving. Garnish with sliced Spanish olives, as desired.

Conclusion

Your oral health has an effect on more than just your teeth. Poor oral and dental health can contribute to issues with your self-esteem, speech, or nutrition. They can also affect your comfort and overall quality of life. Many dental and oral problems develop without any symptoms.

Seeing a dentist regularly for a checkup and exam is the best way to catch a problem before it gets worse.

Lightning Source UK Ltd.
Milton Keynes UK
UKHW020639100622
404229UK00006B/705